Paleo Diet
Eat Healthy For Longevity

Steven Ballinger

Legal Disclaimer

Table of Contents

Important Insight

Losing weight is a challenge for millions of people each year. Even though more and more people are undertaking fitness events ranging from 5K races to triathlons and marathons, the statistics also show that the West is becoming more overweight with each passing year as well.

The culprits are easy to find. Heading out to a restaurant for dinner? You're likely to get a plate of food that has twice as many calories as you need. It's likely to be loaded with carbs and sodium. You'll push back from the table full, but your body will not benefit much as a result.

Heading to the grocery store? The aisle end caps and the sections in the middle of the store are loaded with processed foods in which we over-indulge.

Add this to the sedentary lifestyle that too many people lead, spending both work and leisure hours seated in front of electronic devices of some kind, and you have a dangerous trend in the West: spiraling obesity for people leading increasingly low levels of activity.

The Paleo Diet hearkens back to the ancient days of history when man was a hunter-gatherer. In general terms, the paleo diet includes foods that he would have eaten: fruits, vegetables, meat, game, fish, and nuts. There are no dairy products or grain-based products in this diet, and there is nothing that is processed.

Can this work for you? It's worked for thousands of others. Take a look at the steps that you need to take to put this to work in your own life.

1: Say goodbye to milk

If you take a look inside most people's kitchens, you will find foods that definitely do not fit inside the Paleo Diet. Some of these foods are permitted on other diets – in fact, some of them are encouraged – but if you want to get results from this plan, you'll want to get rid of several things, and the first is the milk.

Since you were a little kid, people have been probably telling you to drink your milk. But on the Paleo Diet plan, you won't ever have to do it again.

Dairy consumption: A recent trend

According to Dr. Loren Cordain, this whole dairy thing is a recent introduction to the human diet. His research shows that dairy products did not enter the human diet until people started practicing agriculture, so about 10,000 years ago. Before that, people had to eat what they could hunt and gather.

It wasn't until people started farming that they domesticated the animals that produce milk, so people didn't start getting milk, butter, yogurt and cheese from those animals until then. People did incorporate cows and goats into their diet before that time, but it was for the meat – not the milk.

Before the first farmers, no one was eating any dairy products.

10,000 years ago sounds like an incredible amount of time to us. However, it's just a small bit of time on the spectrum of human history. Today, people get about 10 percent of their caloric intake from dairy products. This isn't a huge percentage, but it is significant enough to have an influence on our overall nutrition.

And here's something else to think about: humans are the only species on Earth that consumes milk from another animal as an adult. There is no nutritional need for dairy products that come from different species, either for humans or for other mammals.

The dairy industry spends a ton of money each year advertising its products. One of the most well-known campaign uses "Got Milk?" as its slogan, and it shows a variety of celebrities in print, television and radio ads, all with what looks like a milk mustache on their top lips. The implication is that all of these celebrities are endorsing dairy products, which means that they must be healthy, right?

The purpose of milk is to help young animals grow at a rapid pace, and to permit hormones and other chemicals from their mother's milk enter their systems, priming their immune systems and keeping diseases at bay.

As far as young animals go, this is a vital evolutionary stratagem. However, the same is not the case for adult animals consuming food that was designed for another species – and for the young of that species.

Instead of being nutritionally sound, there is a growing body of research showing that dairy products are actually harmful. Two thirds of the people on Earth cannot drink milk without going through bloating, gas and other digestive issues. Such products as soy milk and almond milk have entered the market to help all of the people who are lactose intolerant or simply don't do well with milk.

If you look at the nutritional content of milk, you'll see it's a blend of protein, fat and carbohydrates. Most of the carbs in milk come from lactose, which is a sugar made of galactose and glucose (two simple sugars).

When we eat or drink ice cream, milk or other dairy foods that are high in lactose, our bodies have to use an enzyme known as lactase in our digestive systems to break the lactose back down into those two simple sugars.

The reason why two thirds of the world has problems with lactose is that those people do not have the genetic makeup to produce lactase, and so they cannot tolerate lactose.

You might be thinking that two thirds sounds high. If that's true, you must be from Europe or North America. Northern Europeans and their descendants genetically have high lactase activity in their digestive tracts, which means they can drink milk without any fuss.

However, once you get away from white people and look at Asians, people of African descent and Hispanics, the numbers get a lot higher when it comes to people who can't process dairy in the right way.

But what about people who can process lactase without any problem? The truth is that the nutritional value in milk is still negligible. If you compare milk to the foods in the Paleo Diet (fresh vegetables, seafood, lean meats, fresh fruits, nuts and seeds), what you will discover is that the other food groups are a much better source of Vitamin D as well as other key nutrients that the Western diet tends to lack. Depending on whom you ask, the right amount of Vitamin D per day ranges between 600 and 1000 IU.

If you drink a glass of raw milk, you get 3.6 IU. The fact that dairy processors add Vitamin D to their milk means that a glass will give you 100 IU. You still have to drink six to eight glasses; if you're drinking whole milk, that's 1,680 calories, or about 75 percent of your ideal intake for the whole day.

Some researchers suggest as many as 2000 IU, which means you would have to drink 20 glasses and take in 5,600 calories. Instead of pounding all that milk, all you have to do is step outside and take in some sunlight.

If you consider the role that dairy products can have in terms of heart disease and insulin resistance, the case against milk becomes stronger. Should your children drink milk?

The case among pediatricians is still strong, as it does promote growth, and for infants, breastfeeding is a definite shield against disease. However, for older children, adolescents and adults, there is a growing body of research indicating that it's time to stop drinking milk.

So once you've gotten rid of your milk, you're ready to get rid of some other items in your fridge and pantry that are not part of the Paleo Plan. Read on to learn more!

2: Time to purge the fridge and pantry

Now that the milk is gone, it's time to get rid of those other foods in your house that are not on the Paleo Diet.

This picture probably looks like everything you think you're supposed to eat on a diet. The blueberries are rich in antioxidants, and the strawberries are great as well. However, it's that creamy white stuff – the yogurt – that's not on the Paleo Diet.

That's right – even the nonfat, low-calorie sort of yogurt is not on your list of foods to eat. Just like you're not supposed to drink milk, you don't eat cheese, yogurt, or any other dairy foods. The arguments are the same; the nutritional benefits from dairy foods are more readily available in other food groups, and with less of an impact in terms of calories and fat.

Breads and grains

If you think about what people ate during the Paleolithic time period, it makes sense that bread and grains would not be on this list. After all, bread and grains are agricultural by-products.

This means that people didn't even know that they were a food until the advent of agriculture – again, about 10,000 years ago. Since that time, grains have become a major staple in diets all over the planet. However, there's plenty of good reason to throw out the bread and the pasta.

By this time, you may be ready to delete this e-book and run to the next diet plan. First we tell you to punt your dairy (including that creamy Greek yogurt your trainer told you to eat), and now we're telling you to get rid of grains – especially the whole grains. Stick with us, though, and we'll explain how all of this works.

When the human genetic code was put together, grains were nowhere near being on the radar for the human diet. When we added grains in, we added a food that is chemically different from the foods we were used to eating. Today, though, if you look at the USDA food pyramid, you can see that we are supposed to get between six and eleven servings of grains each day. However, that is terrible advice.

Why do governments want you to eat grains? They are inexpensive to make, you can store them for a lot longer than you can fresh foods, and you can sell them to other countries with a minimum of logistical fuss. For a country like the United States, that has a whole section of the land devoted to grains, these are compelling reasons. After all, exports of grain are great for the American economy.

One of the main nutritional problems that grains present is that they upset the balance of insulin in the body. Our top health problem as a society is elevated insulin levels. The purpose of insulin is to keep blood sugar levels at a healthy range.

When you take in any form of sugar, including carbohydrates, the body generates insulin to bring the levels back low again. When your body has so much sugar that the insulin can't deal with it all, it stores the remainder is fat. If your insulin levels are always high (meaning that you're constantly taking in a lot of sugar), your body undergoes inflammation, and your cells start resisting the work of insulin.

This starts a vicious cycle, as the pancreas has to start shooting out more and more insulin. When your body resists insulin strongly enough, you become diabetic.

In the Western diet, the primary source of carbohydrates is grains (wheat, rice, oats, rye, corn, barley and so on). Pastas and breads come from grain – primarily wheat. Without grains in the diet, it would be a lot harder for people to become fat and develop high levels of insulin. The recommended daily consumption level for carbohydrates is 300 grams. You would have to eat a ton of fruits and vegetables to get that high.

However, if you open that fridge or pantry, you're likely to see sources of carbs that are grain-based all over the place. Do you have bread? Pasta? Rice? How about breakfast cereal? Do you have some leftover birthday cake? How about a box of crackers? These are all staples in the Western diet, and people consume these at a high rate.

So it's time to get rid of these grain-based items out of your refrigerator and your pantry.

Processed foods

If you have a question as to whether something is on the Paleo Diet, take a look at the package. First of all, if it comes in a package, it's probably not on the diet. It likely has a grain base (think meal helpers, boxes of macaroni and cheese and so on). The most likely Paleo Diet foods come in a similar form to what our ancestors would bring home from a day of looking for food.

What about snacks with a "healthy" label like protein bars? They don't have carbs, right?

The truth is that the vast majority of packaged, processed foods have a grain basis that is not going to square with the Paleo Diet plan. Even bars that emphasize protein are not part of the plan.

Think about it this way. If you start with raw ingredients and develop your own meals, you control the levels of sodium, because you're the one adding the seasoning. You control the amount of carbohydrates, because you're not adding sweeteners to build flavor. These are foods that will be on the Paleo Diet plan.

Now that you have lots of packaged food in the trash (or at least in a bag that you will take down to the local food pantry), you're ready to go shopping. You'll be surprised how easy it is to shop – you'll spend a lot less time at the store than you used to. You'll also be more enthusiastic about the meals you're going to make.

Go on to Chapter 3 to learn how to shop for the Paleo Diet.

3: Time to head to the store

Now that you don't have anything to eat, it is time to go shopping. If you don't have food at home to cook, you're likely to eat out, which means that you're going to be eating unhealthy food. Eating at restaurants means you're going to get entrees that are twice as full of calories, carbs and sodium as you need (if not more so), but let's face it – we're all human.

If you get home at the end of the day and the pantry is empty, you're not likely to run out and shop, and then come home and cook. Instead, you're going to head out to eat. If you've been on the Paleo Diet for a few days, that basket of bread sticks is going to look awfully good.
(By the way, if you have non-Paleo food now and then, that's not going to be the end of the world. That's part of the 80% rule. But more about that later).

For now, it's time to get out a sheet of paper and make a list of the things that you want to eat off this list. Many beginners to the Paleo Diet have used this list as a starting point on their journey toward weight loss and better health.

Fresh Produce (that's in Season!)

First of all – not everything in the produce aisle is on the Paleo Diet. Foods that are based in starch, such as white potatoes or corn, need to stay out of your basket. However, you can have just about all of the berries and fruits you want. If you're really trying to maximize weight loss, stay away from the fruits that are especially high in sugar, such as grapes, tangerines and bananas.

When it comes to vegetables, there are seven that you can keep in your crisper twelve months out of the year. They're always sin season, and they're always great accompaniments to a meal when you're on the Paleo Diet. These are: sweet potatoes, bell peppers (all colors), mushrooms, avocados, cabbage (green and purple), broccoli and cauliflower, and any leafy greens (especially kale and spinach).

Meat, meat, meat

So far, this e-book has mostly been about things you CAN'T eat. Well, if you're a big fan of grilled meat, chicken, pork, seafood and other delectable things, you'll love this diet. You can eat eggs (the real thing, not egg whites).

You can have beef (stick with lean cuts and try to get grass-fed, as you won't be getting carbs from the cattle feed). You can have chicken and pork (ideally pasture-fed, for the same reason as with the beef). You can have seafood too, especially that has been caught in the wild.

Check the labels, though. If you come across something that has received antibiotics, nitrates, hormones or other artificial treatment, put it back. It isn't necessarily a nutritional problem, but those are toxins you just don't need to have to deal with.

Fats

I know what you're thinking right now – why on earth would a book about a DIET tell me to go by FAT at the store?

Here's the deal – when you get rid of the majority of carbs in your diet, you gradually start teaching your body to burn fat for energy. This means that you can consume fat without worrying about it being stored in your body, because you will burn it for energy.

Also, there are some fats that your body actually needs in order to be healthy. Ever heard of the Omega-3 family of fatty acids? You'll find these in olive oil and in fish like salmon. They boost the levels of "good" (HDL) cholesterol in your body, and you definitely want them in your diet.

So you definitely want to pick up a bottle of olive oil, as well as some coconut oil. If you shop at a store that sells ghee (clarified butter, which you make by boiling butter and taking out solid milk pieces), then get some.

You definitely want to stay away from canola oil, soybean oil, margarine and any hydrogenated oils. Those will elevate the "bad" (LDL) cholesterol levels in your body.

Nuts

One of the most vulnerable times of day for Paleo Diet eaters is the between-meals snack. If you have a vending machine in your break room, it's unlikely that you'll find things like a small portion of grilled salmon, a raw apple or a quick omelet inside. Instead, you'll find things like potato chips, puffy cheese snacks, and chocolate bars.

The only thing you're likely to find in there that is Paleo friendly is a small back of peanuts, salted to the point where you'll be sprinting over to the soda machine when you are halfway through.

Just about every edible nut you will find is on the list of Paleo Diet foods. It is true that some nuts are higher in fat than others, but remember that you're training your body to use fats instead of sugars as fuel. So go to the grocery store and pick up a variety of nuts: walnuts, almonds, pecans, even some of the higher-fat ones like cashews.

When you're feeling that craving between meals, grab a handful or two, chew them slowly, and then get back to whatever you were doing. You'll be surprised how filling they are.

Following these techniques when you're at the grocery store will help you change your habits as time goes by. After all, you can't eat what you don't have, and if you replace the processed foods, grains and dairy with these healthy alternatives, your habits (and even your cravings) will alter over the course of time. You'll feel better, you'll look better, and your energy levels will be off the charts.

4: Your First Month

For the purposes of this book, I'm assuming that you're leading a fairly sedentary lifestyle and need as much of an overhaul in your exercise program as you do in your diet. The only sort of weight loss that takes place quickly happens when you are dropping water weight; after that is gone, you hit a plateau and start inching back upward. You're making changes for the long haul, so use the first 30 days on the Paleo Diet plan to get accustomed to your new habits.

During this first month focus on three things: adding walking to your lifestyle, getting your sleep patterns set and moving your diet over to the point where you are living Paleo.
How far should you walk? How frequently should you walk? As often as you have some free time, get up out of the chair and get out for a walk, and go until you're tired or until you're out of time. Unless walking is keeping you from sleeping (or eating), you're not walking too much.

If you're already doing a normal cardio routine, drop back and walk. We are genetically programmed to move for long periods of time at relatively low intensity. Get your body used to that habit before you ramp things back up.

If you're not sleeping enough, or you're sleeping at the wrong times of the day, it will be difficult to lose weight. Research shows that you will build up insulin resistance if you don't have the right sleep patterns.

When this happens, your body has a harder time breaking into that stored fat to get energy. If you're not getting the right amount of sleep, you can expect to have more cravings for the wrong types of food, as well as inflammation throughout your body.

These can both cause you to store more fat. What's your goal? Eight hours of sleep a night, ideally between about
10:00 PM and 6:00 AM.

So what should a day or week look like during that first month? Here's one example of what a typical schedule could look like.

Weekday Schedule

- 6:00 AM - Wake up, head out for a 30-minute walk

- 6:30 AM - Breakfast: scrambled eggs with sliced tomatoes, lightly salted

- Get ready for work/commute to office

- 10:00 AM - Get up from your computer and take a 10-minute walk around the office or outside if possible

- 10:10 AM Snack - handful of almonds and a handful of
  baby carrots

- 11:00 AM - Take a 5- to 10-minute walk around the office or outside if possible

- 12:00 PM Lunch - Boneless skinless chicken breast and steamed spinach leftover from dinner the night before, one small to medium sized apple

- 1:00 PM - 5 to 10-minute walk
  Repeat the walks every hour

- 5:30 PM - Arrive home from work, take a 15-minute walk (leash up your dog if you have one – he'll love getting out!)

- 6:00 PM Dinner - Pork chops, applesauce (no sugar added) and steamed broccoli. Portion things right: half of the plate should be filled with broccoli, and the pork and fruit should take up the other half.

- 8:00 PM - Take a 15-20 minute walk

- 10:00 PM - Time for bed

Weekend Day

- 7:00 AM Wake up

- 7:15 AM Breakfast - Frittata with eggs, asparagus, mushrooms and other vegetables as desired (but no cheese!)

- 8:00 AM - Take a hike that lasts several hours. If your town has a state park close by or another attractive hiking venue, this is a great day to visit. Bring some Paleo-friendly snacks with you: fresh fruit and nuts. There are some trail mixes that are Paleo friendly.

- 12:00 PM Lunch - Have some lean protein, such as grilled chicken or salmon, with leafy greens and some fresh fruit. If you want to have a 20% meal on this day (this is one of the meals where you allow yourself to have carbohydrates), this is a good time to do it, because your metabolic level will be elevated somewhat from your long exercise. Make sure to return to Paleo friendly foods for your afternoon snack and for your dinner, and make sure that you get in bed by 10:00 or 11:00.

By the end of your first month, if you've forced yourself to walk frequently and regularly, your body should be champing at the bit for a little more in the way of exercise. If you've stuck faithfully to the eating plan, then the idea of a piece of cake or a slab of deep dish pepperoni pizza may be losing its appeal to you. The body is slow to change, but once change comes, the body adopts its new habits.

You will start to crave the food you've been eating, rather than the food you haven't been eating. If your sleep patterns have become more regular, and you've been getting those eight hours (or more) each night, then you should look more rested and more peaceful when you head out the door each day. Your stores of energy should be increasing; while you are ready to go to sleep at 10 or 11 at night now, you should be feeling fewer lulls throughout the day.

Remember when you used to start nodding off at your desk every day at about 2:00 in the afternoon, even though you'd been pounding diet soda with caffeine throughout the morning and you'd had a hearty lunch? The fact that you are taking in fewer carbs means that your body is not riding that glucose roller coaster every day, cycling between having too much sugar and having your body send insulin into your system.

Instead, your body sugar is moving on a much more reliable continuum, with lower bursts when you get sugar from fruit rather than from breads or other processed foods. That gentler continuum means better health for you.

5: Your Second Month

As you move from your first month into your second on the Paleo Diet, your body is ready for a more advanced progression of changes. The first starts with your carbs.

This is a good time to talk about the Rule of 80%. What this means is that if you can follow the Paleo Diet (or any diet that restricts a particular type of food) 80% of the time, then you are going to get results that are about the same as they would be if you followed it 100% of the time.

What does this mean for you? It means that there are going to be days when you can have some pizza for dinner or a waffle with your breakfast, without seeing your weight ballooning back up as a result.

This way you can build in some meals that involve your very favorite foods, as long as you remember that you can only have these items once every five meals. Outside of that, you need to stick to the Paleo Diet plan.

With this in mind, it's time to start making some refinements. First, cut your consumption of starchy fruits and other similar carbs back. Ultimately, you want your carbs to come from fibrous veggies, at least as much as possible.

Are you a woman? It might be time to analyze your caloric intake, because it's likely that you are not getting enough calories each day.

It's important to keep adequate nutrition so that you can perform the exercise regimen that you want. If you fall below 1800 calories per day, you can suffer a number of other health issues that don't creep up when you're getting enough food.

But what if you're not hungry? Swap more fat into your diet so that your meals and snacks are more filling. Also add to your walking regimen, because the more you walk, the happier you will be.

These changes may feel artificial at first, opposed diametrically to your prior habits. It's all right if you feel like you're not quite yourself; as long as you can work your calories up over time, you'll be ahead of the game.

This is a good time to sing the praises of red meat. You don't want to eat a fatty cut, but you do want the high caloric density of red meat. So look for bison and any variety of beef that is grass fed.

If you have made a habit of allowing yourself too little food, you will add a little bit of fat at first, because your body isn't used to getting what it needs to thrive, and it will hoard some fat at first.

Don't get upset when this happens. Remember, you have to teach your body so that it won't hoard away every bit of fat that comes in the door. Over time, your body will learn to trust you, knowing that you will eat more fat later, so it is safe to burn the fat that you just ate now.

This is the irony of enforced dieting over time. Your body gets used to so little coming in that every tidbit of fat that you eat gets stored somewhere on your body. So while you might be able to work your way down to a weight plateau, every binge will send you back up, and you have so few calories coming in that going to the gym simply is not going to happen, because you won't have the energy to make it through a basic routine.

While cutting your food intake down to the bone (no pun intended) is one way to keep your weight low, it is not a way to manage your health over time. Your levels of key vitamins and other nutrients will sag toward low points, and you will develop other health problems as a result.

As you make your way into your second month, you're going to add weight training to your walking regimen. At least three days a week, you're going to head to the gym to focus on such large compound strength training moves as presses, deadlifts and squats.

You're trying to boost your physical capacity and strength. You're going to get to the point where you can lift significantly more than an average person of your gender and age.

At that point, you may decide to move over to a maintenance program. If this is your first foray into heavy lifting, you need a trainer to show you the right way to lift weight. It's one thing to read a manual about weightlifting form, and it's another to watch videos about how to do it.

But until you have a coach showing you the best in terms of form and showing you in the gym the right way to do it, you won't get the most out of strength training.

If you sign up at a recreation center in your town, or at a private gym, you can get a referral to a trainer who will help you. Let the management know that you are on the Paleo Diet and want exercises that are compatible with your nutritional plan.

The management at the gym or private fitness club will be able to connect you with someone who will help you. No matter who ends up training you, though, make sure you learn all about form and mobility.

You don't want to hurt yourself three months into your weightlifting career; instead, you want to be lifting weights twenty years from now, so learn the right form and use it to start building toward the results that you want. Remember that walking and heavy lifting will combine to help you burn more fat than simple cardio over time.

If you haven't done so in the past, consider meditation as a way to build mental focus. There are quite a few different methods that work. This is not necessarily spiritual in nature, so you should be able to develop a level of comfort with it even if you are agnostic or an atheist.

This is just a way to manage the stress in your life. Try it faithfully for a couple of weeks, and you are sure to enjoy the effects it has on you physically, emotionally and mentally.

Why meditation? Remember that our genes lead all the way back to ancient times. When we received our genetic code as a species, the world was a significantly different place. Modern society involves stresses that differ significantly from what we were evolved to encounter.

We are programmed to fight battles, to hunt down food, to conquer tangible difficulties in our way. Instead, we are dealing with making mortgage and car payments, kowtowing to bosses who are simply more stress than they are worth, and sitting in traffic while wondering whether or not the sprinkler system will turn on on the right day.

These so-called "emergencies" have just about no bearing on our survival, but they engender a response in the body that is quite similar to the stress of survival. Instead of coming all at once, though, this stress response happens slowly, over a long time. Meditation is one of the few practices that work for just about everyone in that situation.

6: Months 3 and 4

In your third month, you won't need to make any changes to your diet. You should already be free of grains, pasta and dairy, as well as most processed foods, at least 80 percent of the time, and you still should be focused on getting your carbs from the less sugary fruits and vegetables.

However, it is time to ramp up your exercise plan. You added some weight training in Month 2, so now you're going to add some interval workouts. These involve alternating between intense bursts of activity and periods of rest.

An example could be going to a track and alternating between jogging and sprinting, such as jogging on the curves of the track and sprinting on the straight sections. You can also do this on a rowing machine or on a stationary bike. The key is hitting 100% effort for 20 or 30 seconds at a time.

Adding anywhere between three and five sprints to your workout to start is a good plan. Make sure, though, that you begin with walking and light cycling or jogging before you get into the intense workout. Also, once you are finished, stretching is a must to keep you from experiencing an injury.

Once you get into your fourth month, analyze your progress and see if you are losing fat. If you want to be technical about this, you can go to a trainer and have a body fat analysis performed. This will tell you what your percentage of body fat is.

If you are losing fat, simply keep following the habits you already have, as you are on the way to long-term weight loss and fat loss that will improve your life dramatically. However, if you are not losing fat yet, there are some more changes that you can make at this point to help you make progress.

One change is known as Intermittent Fasting. This refers to consolidating all of your caloric consumption into a shorter time frame during the day. Some people refer to this as the "Eight Hour Diet," and all it means is that you take in all of your calories during an eight-hour window during the day.

You don't want to cut your caloric consumption, because you want to keep your metabolic activity high. However, you do want to get all of your calories in during a particular time frame. One of the easiest ways to do this is to eat between 11:00 AM and 7:00 PM.

It is true that many dietary experts suggest that breakfast is vital; if you find that your metabolism really tails off if you skip breakfast, think about a window between 9:00 AM and 5:00 PM. For most people, going without an evening meal is not realistic, because of social obligations and family habits. However, moving dinner a little bit earlier should not cause that much of an inconvenience.

Another change has to do with the calories you are taking in. If your appetite is considerable and you are still taking in a lot of calories, it may be time to adjust that count downward. If you are exercising regularly and are a woman, you need between 1800 and 2000 calories at minimum; if you are a man, you need between 2200 and 2400 calories.

If you are eating more than that, though, it's time to bring it downward if you are not losing fat yet. Sometimes just bringing those calories down a bit can trigger fat loss. However, you don't want to cut so much out that you start losing muscle mass.

If your body thinks that it is going through starvation, it will start consuming muscle for food, and when you start burning muscle, your metabolism goes down as well.

Finally, you can start cycling the way in which you take in carbs. One way to do this is to stick with 30 grams or less in carbs on most days, but giving yourself high starch content in a couple of dinners per week, in the form of butternut squash, yams or white rice, your body is likely to start shedding fat, because the carb cycling convinces your body that you don't intend to starve it.

In the next chapter, I put together a Paleo Diet eating plan to follow for two weeks. Preparing food for this sort of lifestyle requires some prior planning, but you'll be surprised how easily you are able to put together a plan that works for you.

It does take some discipline (after all, it's always easier to roll through a drive through window or call and order pizza than it is to prepare a healthier alternative). You will love the new life that you have simply because of how much better you will feel.

7: Two Weeks in the Paleo Life

Here is a sample meal plan for you to follow as you make your way through your week. If you shop for this on Sundays, you'll be surprised at how easy it is to stick with it. Just stick it up on your refrigerator, so you'll know what you're eating.

Day	Breakfast	AM Snack	Lunch	PM Snack	Dinner
1	3-egg omelet Veggies of choice Fried in coconut oil	Celery w/ Nut butter	Tuna salad in a lettuce wrap w/avocado	Green tea	Steak with mushrooms w/ small spinach salad
2	Meat (4-6 oz) with ¼ cup of nuts of choice	2 hardboiled eggs, handful of berries	Salad w/ grilled chicken, vinaigrette of olive oil and lemon juice	Green tea	Pork chops, onions, sautéed zucchini, mushrooms
3	2-3 eggs fried in coconut oil, ½ avocado	Celery w/ nut butter	2 beef patties with a fresh tomato and ½ avocado	Green tea	CHEAT MEAL (gluten free)
4	Pork sausage 1-2 cups cooked green veggies	2-3 oz beef jerky with handful of berries	Club sandwich in a lettuce wrap with mayo	Green tea	Roast beef, small spinach salad, steamed broccoli
5	2-3 hardboiled eggs, ½ avocado, pork sausage	¼ cup nuts	4-5 salmon patties with steamed broccoli	Green tea	Sausage and pepper sautee, with spices and spinach
6	Bacon and eggs with grapefruit	Raw vegetables with guacamole	Steak salad with caramelized onions and sun-dried tomatoes,	Green tea	Bowl of chili, small salad with olive oil dressing

			garlic, olive oil and balsamic vinaigrette		
7	Scramble of leftover meat and eggs	2-3 ounces of beef jerky w/ handful of berries	Mexican chili salad	Green tea	Salmon with mashed cauliflower and asparagus
8	2 poached eggs, ½ cup chili, green tea		Chicken with fried mushrooms and zucchini	Paleo cookies or muffins	4 oz curried salmon fillet on spinach salad
9	3 oz salmon, ½ cup broccoli, green tea		Leftovers (finish the fresh produce, tossing in a pan with a protein, herbs and spices		Rotisserie chicken stir fry
10	3 mini quiches with green tea		Chicken basil salad	2 pieces of 75% dark chocolate with ¼ cup of almonds	CHEAT MEAL
11	2 hardboiled eggs ¼ avocado 1 tomato Green tea		Garlic shrimp salad with 1 cup of raw vegetables	Frozen or fresh blueberries with ¼ cup sliced almonds	Roast beef with turnip and fried beets w/ small salad
12	2 pancakes with green tea and berries		Chicken Caesar salad	Celery and carrot sticks with almond butter	Steak and mushrooms with asparagus
13	Veggie omelet with 2 slices of bacon		CHEAT MEAL		Chili on spinach salad
14	Veggie omelet with 2 slices of bacon		Spinach salad with 4 oz protein (fish or chicken)	Homemade trail mix	Steak with steamed broccoli

Here are some things to remember. When there is a CHEAT MEAL, this means that you can eat whatever you want (except for the gluten-free meal in the first week). Have you been craving some spaghetti? Wanting a piece of pie? This is the time to do it. However, remember that the formula for weight loss is still the same: the more calories you take in, the more calories you have to burn in order to lose weight. So enjoy yourself, but be reasonable.

A lot of the meals on this plan sound like they might require a great deal of preparation. However, there are some ways that you can work those meals into a busy day without driving yourself into the ground by cooking after a work day. One example has to do with chili.

You can put the ingredients for chili into a slow cooker before you head out the door for work, and it will cook while you are gone. When you get home, you will walk in the door to the delicious smell of chili – and it will be ready for you to eat.

The same goes for meats like roast beef and roasted chicken. You can cook these in a slow cooker throughout the day as well, pulling them out when you get home. There are some recipes that allow you to cook the vegetables inside the cooker as well, meaning you have a complete meal ready when you get home.

Also, you can cook multiple portions at the same time, dividing the food into different containers that you can freeze and then thaw out when it is time for that particular meal.

You may have noticed that the snacks dwindle in the second week. The longer you are in the Paleo Diet, the more accustomed your body becomes to a decreased level of carbohydrates.

As your blood sugar levels even out, going through fewer and fewer spikes, you will find that your cravings during the middle of the morning and early afternoon become less pressing. The need for the morning snack should go away entirely, and you'll find that you need less in the afternoon as well.

The reason for this is that when you are on a carb-based diet, your body ebbs and flows between cycles of sugar intake and insulin correction, as your body seeks to regulate the amount of sugar in the bloodstream. The need for snacks comes from the "sugar crash" in your system.

When you are on the Paleo Diet, you don't have the insulin leaning on your blood sugar totals, and so you don't have the constant need to put more food into the system.

When you do have meals, remember that you can have just about all the vegetables you want. So if you finish your plate (remember, half veggies, half proteins and carbs) and still want more, you can go back and get more veggies. Also, remember that if you eat more slowly at each meal, you will find them more filling.

8: Tips for Beginning

Do you feel like all this is a little too much to take on at once? That's all right – you are not alone. Take a look at some tips that you can try one at a time. Maybe you can think about adding them to your lifestyle, one each day. As you start to feel better, you may want to add them more quickly.

1. Get rid of food groups one at a time. Instead of dumping sugars, dairy, beans and grains all at once, think about getting rid of a different group every week.

2. When you're ready to purge, purge the processed foods all at once. This might mean getting out one of this big lawn and leaf bags to get the job done.

3. Start with one meal at a time. Instead of jumping into the full menu, begin by going to Paleo snacks. Then move to dinner, and lunch, and then breakfast, changing a different meal each week. Breakfast generally has the most carbs (cereal, toast, waffles,

pancakes, and so on), so that may be the toughest to dislodge.

4. Can't work a meal at a time? Instead, focus on getting one non-paleo item out of your diet at a time. Maybe you're having a hard time staying away from pizza of French fries. Figure out which of these applies to you, and pick one. You'll notice that you crave each one less as time goes by, and you will slowly build up positive momentum.

5. Can't stand the idea of throwing all the bad food out at once? Make your transition gentler by simply shopping differently. Instead of throwing out that big bag of Wavy Lays, make that your last bag. When you go to the store, replace it with snacks that are on the Paleo list. This will keep you from feeling like you are wasting money as well.

6. Prepare, prepare, prepare. If you try and copy the two-week meal list from this e-book and use it every week, you will burn out quickly, because you'll tire of the same foods. Keep

the cheat meals at roughly the same intervals, but keep finding more and more meals that you can use. You'll enjoy broadening your palate and finding new ways to prepare proteins and vegetables in a tasty way.

7. Don't beat yourself up if you slip up in the early phases. C.S. Lewis said that eating is just a biological act. If you mess up, you will slow down your progress a bit. However, one meal is not the end of the world; if you go ahead and call that your cheat meal, then you can make up for it later that week. Even if you have an extra cheat meal or two, you're still making progress. The stress from beating yourself up is likely to push you to go back to your old eating habits, so the less stress, the more success.

8. Get everyone in your house on the same menu. Admittedly, this will be hard, because you're not going to be the only one who doesn't like giving up carbs. However, giving different family members the chance to plan the cheat meals, and the slow progress of

feeling healthier as a family, will make this something you will be glad you did.

9. Think about starting with a weeklong juice fast instead of being gradual. If you're going to have sugar cravings and withdrawals for your favorite foods, you might as well go big and begin with a juice fast. That way, the foods on the Paleo Diet will seem like a reward rather than an awful regimen. You'll also be starting your new eating plan with those withdrawals behind you.

10. Don't ever, ever, ever use the word diet. This is a word that sounds like the complete opposite of fun, in the first place. You see it stamped on cans and bottles of soda that don't taste very good, bottles of juice that don't have much flavor, and processed snacks that come in portions that are too small and that taste like Styrofoam.

Also, diets sound temporary. People go on diets until they lose that desired amount of weight, and then they come off them. Too often, though, the weight comes back on. Why? Because once the diet is over, people think they can go back to their old ways of eating. They shouldn't be surprised, then, when that weight returns, because their old habits are back.

Instead, focus on the idea of a lifestyle change. You're not doing something for a few weeks or a few months. Instead, you're changing the way that you live, and you're going to keep those changes in place permanently.

You're going to be healthier, have more energy, live longer and have a higher quality of life. Thinking about going Paleo in those terms makes it easier to stay motivated.

Use these ten tips to get your mind in order so that you are ready for the coming changes. They will be hard, but you can work through them, and you'll be glad you did.

9: Building a New Mindset

Now that the word "diet" is on its way out of your vocabulary, it's time to think about the new life that you're building for yourself. This starts by creating a whole new way of thinking, so that you stay motivated to stick with the Paleo plan, even on the days when you smell pizza everywhere you go and just HAVE to have a slice.

You don't have to hypnotize yourself, but you do need to change your way of thinking.

Focus on the rewards that this change will bring

Just about everyone wants to lose weight. However, once the cravings hit, or once they hit a plateau, many people simply give up and return to their former ways. Instead of focusing on the number on the scale, or the number you receive when you get your body fat screening, think about the things you'll be able to do once you've made this lifestyle change.

Are you thinking about losing 50 pounds? You're almost there, but that's a goal that may end up frustrating you. What if you lose 10 and plateau then? A lot of people end up quitting. Instead, think of an activity that you will be able to do.

When your kids go to the playground, can you play with them? Or is walking to the park and making it to the bench the best you can do?

One of your best friends is raising money for the Leukemia & Lymphoma Society through Team in Training, and she is going to run a half-marathon at the end of her training season. A half-marathon might sound like a trip all the way around the world right now, but wouldn't it be fun to try a 5K?

When you were a kid, your parents took you to hike part of the Appalachian Trail. Wouldn't it be fun to be able to take your own kids there and recreate that family tradition?

Aren't you tired of getting home from work and having just enough energy to change into some comfortable clothes and slouch down in front of the television? Wouldn't it be great to have the energy to play a family board game, take your kids for a bike ride around the park, or hop on your bike for 10 or 15 miles before dinner?

When you're standing in line at the grocery store, you see all of those articles about spicing up your love life at home. Even though you love your spouse, you just don't have the energy to get things going anymore. Wouldn't it be great to feel just as sexy as the people on the covers of those advice magazines?

These are just some of the rewards that await you when you improve your health and energy levels. Think about one or all of these when you're a few weeks in to the Paleo eating plan and you're sick and tired of steamed broccoli.

Understand that it is all right not to be perfect

It's one thing to tape a meal plan on the refrigerator. It's quite another to live that plan out, a day at a time, until you hit the end. Even when you have your handful of nuts and berries ready to go for a mid-morning snack on a particular Thursday, you might see a box of donuts in the break room at work, or some leftover pizza on your co-worker's desk with a sign on it that says, "Help yourself!"

All of a sudden, you find yourself scarfing down carbs, and you weren't supposed to have a cheat meal for three more days.

For many of us, the natural solution is to get angry at ourselves and tell ourselves that we will never, ever meet our goals. This can turn into a cycle of low self-esteem that ends up pushing us right back to our old culinary friends – things like pizza buffets, large pieces of cake, heaping bowls of ice cream.

The carbs and fats in these types of food are briefly soothing, but then going back to them turns into a cycle that keeps repeating itself. Those five pounds you lost at the start of your Paleo program? Now you've gained ten as a result.

Here's the deal – it's all right if you have a meal that isn't Paleo (isn't even close!) at a time when you don't have "CHEAT MEAL" on the calendar. You're human, and you're going to have off days. As long as you don't let those off days become off weeks, you're going to be all right. The key is to remember that everyone goes through struggles like this, and that you can make permanent change.

So if you find yourself at the bottom of a bowl of ice cream you know wasn't on your list, instead of beating yourself up, lick the bottom of the bowl. Enjoy what you just ate – after all, ice cream is good for a reason. At your next workout, add ten or fifteen minutes of effort. When you have your next meal, have exactly what the Paleo calendar says you are supposed to have. It's all right to fall down, but you have to get right back up.

Keep things as easy as possible

It's hard enough to make lifestyle changes when you don't have any other issues going on in your life. When you have several kids to shuttle around from one activity to the other, when you have stress in the workplace, when your aging parents are making more and more demands on you, it is hard to remember that you're supposed to take care of yourself too.

When it comes to living the Paleo plan for eating, make your life as easy as possible. Get to know how to work your slow cooker. When you go shopping, pick the vegetables out that you like the best. Is there cauliflower on your plan, but you hate cauliflower? Make a substitution.

This is YOUR plan for success. On Sunday afternoons, make some of your dinners and then throw them in the freezer. This plan is supposed to make your life better, not turn it into drudgery. Make this as easy as you can.

10: Yes, Paleo Is a Great Way to Live

Remember a few chapters ago when we said that you need to eliminate the word "diet" from your vocabulary? We meant it. This is a lifestyle that you can enjoy rather than dread, and the time to start doing this is now. Take a look at these tips for making Paleo living something to brag about.

Bacon is awesome

And it's on your list of foods you can eat! Obviously, you don't want to go all bacon, all the time, because lean proteins are your friend as well. However, when you want a slice of bacon or two with your meal, get it out and fry it up. Preferably in some olive oil. You can't have that coconut cake that you love, but you can still have some bacon, so enjoy yourself.

Put the heat into your diet

Did you know that hot sauce is a great way to rev up your metabolism? It's on your list of accepted Paleo condiments as well. So get the bottle of hot sauce out and splash a bit on what you eat. Whether it's scrambled eggs, chili, grilled chicken or shrimp, add a big dose of flavor when you sprinkle some hot sauce on top.

Enjoy your cheat days

We already told you that you need to treasure your goals and keep them in your mind if you want to avoid slipping up on the Paleo plan.

However, when you see that you have a CHEAT MEAL coming up on the calendar, it's all right to think about what you're going to give yourself as a treat at that time. If your mom has an amazing recipe for a meatball, give her a call and invite yourself over for a pasta dinner.

If there is a place that makes handmade ice cream a few blocks away, it's all right to envision that amazing cone a day or two before you get there. The more positivity you have in your system, the easier it is to maintain discipline.

Don't forget the chocolate

Now, you'll want to stay away from the milk chocolate. But dark chocolate (check the packaging to see that it is at least 75% dark chocolate) is good for your heart, and it is on the Paleo list.

You might be thinking that hunters and gatherers didn't bring back chocolate to their huts, but the bottom line is that the health benefits outweigh the disadvantages, so you can definitely add some to your stack of snacks.

Find a deep freezer at a garage sale

Everyone enjoys finding a bargain, so head out to a garage sale or a swap meet to find a deep freezer. This will make your life easier when it comes to preparing and keeping your Paleo meals for the week. When meat goes on sale at the store, you can buy in bulk without worrying that some of it will spoil. Simply throw the meat you're not going to eat for a while into the deep freezer.

Become friends with the hardboiled egg

Yes, you can slice them in half, add some curry powder and mustard, and turn them into deviled eggs. However, this versatile food can become your new snack staple or your new breakfast food when you just don't have time to whip up an omelet or fry a few strips of bacon.

How can you make this easy? On Sunday, boil a dozen eggs, and then put them into a big storage bag in your crisper. Go ahead and peel the shell off. Then, when you're running late for work but really need something for breakfast, grab two or three of them and wrap them in a paper towel.

That way, instead of going through a breakfast drive through and wasting a glorious cheat meal, you have your breakfast sitting right next to you in the car. You'll save money and time in addition to keeping your cheat meal ready for something you'll really enjoy.

Be the snack guy (or girl) at work

When you shop for your weekly Paleo plan, don't just shop for your refrigerator and pantry at home. You never know when those food cravings are going to strike, so you need to be prepared. This means having that can of nuts in the console in your car.

You can't keep pork chops in your desk drawer at work, but you can keep beef jerky. Roast beef won't do so well in your locker, but you can keep a banana or a few apples. If you're really enterprising, you can whip up a batch of trail mix to share with other people when you're hungry.

Making the lifestyle changes that are a part of the Paleo plan is not easy. If it were, you would see a lot fewer obese people walking around. The grip that sugars and processed foods have on our collective willpower is strong, and fighting free of it is a real struggle.

The good news is that you have people who have gone before you and succeeded. If you are ready to see your life change for the better, if you are ready for higher levels of energy, if you are ready to go through a day without riding the sugar roller coaster, it's time to go Paleo. Get started today!

Conclusion

Now that you have finished reading this book, you have access to a set of meal plans, exercises and tips to help you transform your body with the Paleo Diet.

The key to any plan like this is discipline, and new disciplines are difficult to begin – and often even more difficult to maintain.

Remember that the road to transformation is going to be a long one, so be patient with yourself. Allow yourself the freedom to fail from time to time.

As long as you are making progress from week to week and month to month, you will see the changes in your body, and the positive results will turn into a cycle that makes the discipline simpler and simpler to follow. Good luck in your new life!